Stretching Ex
for Over 40

Step-By-Step Guide On How To Get Started With Stretching Exercises For Everyone

Introduction

Are you 40, slightly over 40, or way over 40, and you have recently been thinking of improving your lifestyle and getting fitter?

Have you tried looking for simple stretching exercises for people over 40, and you've come up short?

If so, welcome to the world of stretching exercises!

You probably have seen stretching being done either before a workout or after. But did you know you can do stretching exercises without the workout and still maintain a healthy lifestyle? Yes, you can!

Being 40 and over does not mean that you are doomed, waiting to grow older into an inactive life. If it is what you have believed, then it's time to change your way of thinking.

Stretching exercises can help you slow down the aging process, helping you to continue with your active life, doing the things you love.

Are you excited to start your stretching exercises, but you are wondering where to start?

You may be wondering:

How will the stretch exercises improve your health?

How long should the stretch activities be?

Is stretching the same as warming up?

Are there specific exercises done before and after a workout?

How can you plan an effective routine?

What are the best stretching exercises to start with?

Should you start with a whole-body stretch exercise, or should you start with exercises for specific parts of your body?

Do you need close monitoring when you begin your exercises?

What visible changes will you see as you do stretch exercises?

If you have these and many more questions, then this book is for you.

In this book, you will find:

- **Types of stretch exercises for people over 40.**

- The benefits of stretch exercises.

- **How to plan a stretch exercise routine.**

- Importance of being consistent in your routine program.

- **The difference between warm-ups and stretching exercises.**

- How to avoid possible risks and the safety measures to take as you exercise.

- **The aspects of a good stretch for positive results.**

- When to see a doctor.

- **And much more!**

This book is a guide on how to begin an effective stretching exercise routine. You will know the different types of stretch exercises, the elements of a good stretch, the risks involved, the safety measures to take, and when to see a doctor.

Without further ado, let's get started!

PS: I'd like your feedback. If you are happy with this book, please leave a review on Amazon.

Please leave a review for this book on Amazon by visiting the page below:

https://amzn.to/2VMR5qr

Table of Contents

Introduction 2

Chapter 1: Is Stretching Good For You? 8

    The Benefits of Stretching 12

Chapter 2: Warm-Up or Stretching, Which Comes First? 15

    Types of Warm-Up Exercises 16

Chapter 3: Elements of a Good Stretch 21

Chapter 4: Types of Stretching Exercises- Dynamic Stretching 26

    Dynamic Stretches 26

    How Safe Is Dynamic Stretching For You? 40

Chapter 5: Static Stretching 41

Chapter 6: Ballistic Stretching 54

    Is Ballistic Stretching Safe For You? 55

    Types of Ballistic Stretching 57

Chapter 7: Isometric Stretching 70

Chapter 8: PNF (Proprioceptive Neuromuscular Facilitation) Stretching ..84

Types of PNF Stretching.................................84

Precautions to Take As You Perform PNF Stretches... 88

Chapter 9: How to Start Your Stretching Routine 89

Chapter 10: Safety Tips and Overcoming Risks 99

When to See a Doctor... 101

Conclusion 104

Chapter 1: Is Stretching Good For You?

Why do you need stretch exercises? Are they necessary?

Did you know your muscles are an interesting part of your body that helps you move about and do many things and help your organs function properly? For example, the muscles in your legs help you walk or run, while the muscles in your hands help you lift things.

From the age of 40[1], muscles begin to lose their strength and mass, making one less tolerant to daily activities. If you do not counteract this, you will slowly find normal activities more difficult as you grow older.

Muscles tend to shorten and become tight when they are inactive. That is why if you attempt to carry out strenuous activities, you feel tired and weak, unable to move about with flexibility. This can end up putting your joints at risk of pain and strain, including damage to the muscle.

An exercise regimen is highly recommended to help you maintain your agility for much longer as you age. This is where stretch exercises come in to help you improve

---

[1] https://blog.insidetracker.com/muscles-shrink-as-we-age-fight-back

flexibility, and if you wish, you can add a workout regimen. Otherwise, stretch exercises can also be done on their own and still improve your general health.

Stretching is a form of exercise involving flexing either a specific or a group of muscles to improve muscle tone and elasticity, which results in muscle flexibility, muscle control, and different range of motions. Stretching does more than improve your muscles but also improves your posture, reduces body aches and stress.

You may have noticed a distinct difference between those who exercise and those who do not. It is not a surprise to see people over [60][2] years who are still very active in their daily lives because they have incorporated stretching exercise as part of their lifestyle. It's important to embrace a healthier lifestyle by improving your muscle tone and strength through stretching exercises.

Become a Stronger You!

While hormonal and neurological decline are inevitable changes that happen in your body as you grow older, it is possible to slow down the breakdown of your muscles. The

---

[2] https://blog.insidetracker.com/muscles-shrink-as-we-age-fight-back

cells in the human body are constantly being destroyed and rebuilt to ensure your organs remain strong and function well. If the breaking down of cells outweighs the rebuilding process, then muscle loss begins to set in.

The good news is that muscle degradation can be slowed down through stretch exercises, not forgetting to incorporate a workout plan and a healthy diet. To begin, you need to have a variety of exercises to perform at least three times a week, gradually increasing your exercises as you add more difficult ones, resulting in a stronger you with increased flexibility.

To successfully achieve your goal, commitment is required, and you can do this through the following:

- *Consistency*

Consistency is crucial if you are to see any meaningful results. You will not see any changes in the first few weeks, but you ought to be happy with your outcome in a couple of months. That is why you have to stick to the regimen your trainer sets for you or one that you set for yourself.

- *Correct Execution*

As with any other exercise regimen, you have to do the stretches correctly for them to be effective. Quality of your exercise is more important than quantity; therefore, learn to execute them correctly for maximum results.

The Benefits of Stretching

Below are some of the reasons why you should incorporate stretching into your routine:

1. Increased Flexibility

As you age, you lose your agility, but it can be slowed down by performing stretch exercises.

This could be considered to be the main aim of stretching. It will improve performance in your everyday activities.

2. Range of Motion Is Increased

Moving your joints easily through any range of motion helps you be more active, which improves by stretching regularly. The best stretch exercise for increasing your range of motion is static and dynamic stretches and we will look at both.

PNF (which we will learn about later on in the book) stretching[3] has been proven to be the best stretching technique because it stretches the muscles to your highest limit. More significant gains have been seen through this method.

---

[3] https://www.ncbi.nlm.nih.gov/pmc/articles/PMC3273886/

3. Improved Performance in Physical Activities

Performance in your daily physical activities is improved. If you are an athlete or exercise regularly, you will notice increased performance by stretching regularly.

4. Blood Flow Increase to Your Muscles

When you stretch before a workout, blood flow is increased to your muscles, thereby improving circulation in your body. This means you will be able to recover in a shorter time after a workout than if you did not stretch.

It also reduces muscle soreness after a workout.

5. Improved Posture

Sitting down slumped over your laptop for too long or standing for long hours can distort your posture. Stretching exercises, especially the isometric ones, can strengthen specific muscles, thereby improving your body alignment.

For example, as we will see, planks work on your core muscles to improve posture in your lower and mid-back.

6. Prevents and Heals Back Pain

Lack of exercise makes your muscles become tight and decreases the range of motion in your muscles. You can especially end up straining the muscles in your back, causing a strain that could lead to an injury.

Stretching is an excellent solution to healing your back pain, and through a regular routine, you can also prevent the risk of muscle strain and injury.

7. Great Stress Reliever

When you are stressed, there's a high likelihood that your muscles are tense. This happens because your muscles become tight as a response to emotional and physical stress.

The areas in your body that tend to hold stress the most include the neck, upper back, and shoulders. Therefore these are the areas you should focus on when stretching to relieve stress.

8. Calm Mind

Stretching can help calm your mind, and when coupled with exercises such as meditation, it becomes very effective.

9. Decreases Tension Headaches

Headaches caused by stress and tension can greatly interfere with your daily life. Through plenty of rest, hydration, and a good diet, stretching can help reduce these headaches.

Now, let's get a little into stretching in the next chapter.

Chapter 2: Warm-Up or Stretching ,Which Comes First?

Warm-ups are solely for increasing your body temperature in readiness for a workout. A good warm-up is when the temperature of your body increases between 1.4 to 2.8 degrees Fahrenheit[4].

It is important to warm up before your stretch exercises because it not only loosens stiff muscles if correctly done but improves performance during your workouts. On the other hand, not warming up or doing it incorrectly can increase the likelihood of an injury during your main exercises.

Warm-ups prepare your body for the main workout by increasing your heart rate and blood flow to the rest of your muscles. The warm-up exercises do not have to be complex. You can choose a simple activity that lasts between 5 and 10 minutes.

---

[4]

http://www.edu.xunta.gal/ftpserver/portal/S_EUROPEAS/ED_FISICA2/WARMING_UP.htm

Types of Warm-Up Exercises

Before your workout, you can start with a general warm-up by rotating your joints. You can either begin by rotating your toes and working your way up or from your fingers and downwards.

This aids in joint movement and allows your joints to be lubricated with synovial fluid[5]. The lubrication helps you to move easily during your stretch exercises and workout.

Rotating involves performing circular movements slowly, both clockwise and anticlockwise, and can be done in the following order or in reverse:

1. Toes
2. Ankles
3. Knees
4. Legs
5. Hips
6. Trunk waist

---

[5] https://www.webmd.com/arthritis/synovial-joint-fluid-analysis

7. Neck

8. Shoulders

9. Elbows

10. Wrists

11. Fingers and Knuckles

Let's look at 2 examples of joint rotation:

1. Ankle Rotation

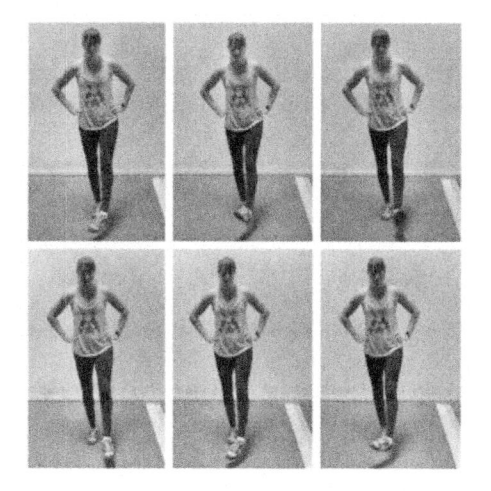

This is a simple exercise that involves your calve and ankle muscles. Start with small circles and progressively increase the diameter to loosen your ankle joints as much as you can. Your flexibility will improve, preventing injuries while you exercise- breathe slowly as you rotate your ankles.

This is one of the recommended warm-ups before working out your lower body. To warm up and increase mobility, a set of 30 moves on each ankle is recommended.

Instructions

1. With your arms by your sides, stand with your feet hip-width apart.

2. With the right leg firmly on the ground, slightly lift your left leg forward and point your toes downwards to the ground.

3. To rotate, make small circles with your left ankle.

4. Repeat with your right foot.

Be careful not to fall over.

2. Leg Rotation

To perform this exercise, you will need to stand with your back straight and your head up, keeping your abs tight. To control your movements, don't bend the leg's knee that is firmly on the ground.

Your goal is to focus on anchoring your body and working fully with your abs. This exercise increases your balance, coordination and builds long, strong, and lean muscles. It's great for your lower body workout, helping to tone your inner thighs, glutes, and quadriceps[6].

You can do between 10 and 15 circles on each leg, starting with small circles, slowly increasing the diameter of your circles. To build more muscle, add ankle weights and do 3 sets, repeating 8 to 12 times.

---

[6] https://www.britannica.com/science/quadriceps-femoris-muscle

Instructions

1. With your arms on your sides, stand straight with feet shoulder-wide apart.

2. Raise one leg almost the height of your knee and rotate it clockwise and then anticlockwise.

3. Switch legs and repeat the motions.

After warming up by rotating your joints, you can then engage in aerobic activity such as skipping rope or jumping for at least 5 minutes. This aims to increase your body temperature in readiness for your stretch exercise and workout as it causes blood to flow to the muscles, hence improving their movement.

Chapter 3: Elements of a Good Stretch

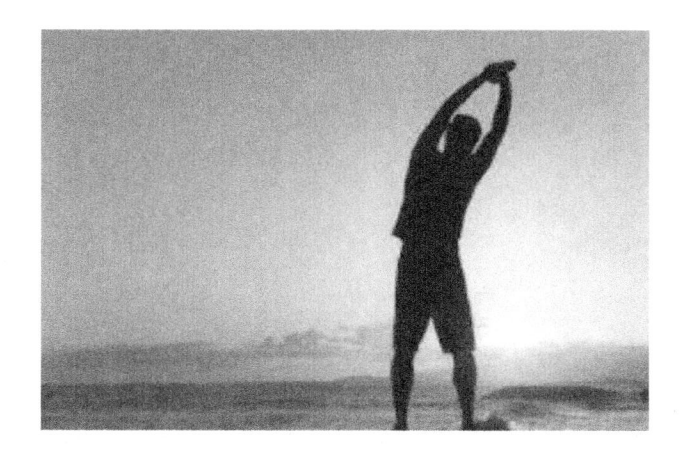

There is a correct way of doing your stretches. If you experience more pain, aches, and cramps, then it's highly likely that you are doing your stretches wrong. Below are some factors to consider when determining the effectiveness of a stretching exercise:

1. Isolation

An effective stretch works only the muscles that need to be stretched. Ideally, your stretch is better if you work fewer muscles at each given time. For example, stretching one hamstring will experience more resistance than stretching both hamstrings at the same time.

This way, you have more control over the stretch, making it easy to increase its intensity. Ensure you pull on your muscle when you stretch.

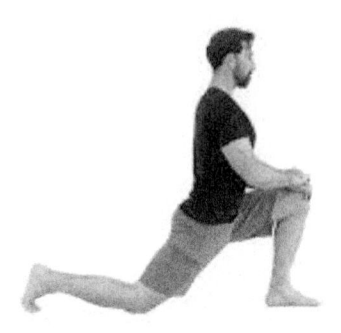

To stretch correctly, you need to pull on your muscle using some force but not too much. For example, when stretching your quadriceps, the best way to do it is to stretch one leg back while you grab the other knee and then stretch.

Do you feel the stretch in your quads? If you do not, then you're not doing it well. You need to feel the pull in your muscle. To do the quad stretches correctly, you need to try and push your quads harder or do different types of moves like kneeling on the floor as your body falls backward. This stretches both your legs at once, and your body weight increases the intensity.

2. Leverage

To leverage on your stretch simply means having control over how intense you want your stretch to be and how fast you can do it. With good leverage, you can achieve the intensity of the stretch that you desire without applying so much force.

Try making your stretches easier and effective by providing greater leverage. Slowly, you will overcome the resistance of your muscles that are difficult to flex.

3. Don't Rush

Never hurry when performing your stretches, especially after you work out, as this could be non-productive. Rushing through a stretch will not give you positive results.

Instead, be as slow as possible, and be still when performing a stretch. For example, if you are doing a neck stretch, don't do it with quick and jerky movements, as you could end up hurting yourself. Also, you will most probably feel sharp pains and more tension, causing your muscle to contract instead of relax.

4. Stretch for The Required Length of Time

You need to time yourself when doing your stretches. Don't hold your stretches for a short time, and neither for too long. Hold each stretch for 30 seconds. It may be difficult initially, but in the end, you will find it easier, and you'll become more flexible.

5. Breathing

Breathing is essential during stretching, as your muscles stretch when you inhale.

For example, breathe in when stretching your triceps as you bend your arm behind your head. Continue breathing as you stretch slowly, pushing your bent arm with your other hand to make it more intense. Exhale slowly as you release your arm, bringing it back to its starting position.

Your muscle relaxes when you exhale, and when you inhale, you lengthen it when stretching.

6. Risk

Despite a stretch being effective through isolation and leveraging, each stretch exercise has the potential risk of an injury. This means you have to consider any possible risk of an injury in each stretch exercise you intend to perform.

An exercise can cause an injury if it puts too much strain on the joints, placing too much stress on the ligaments or tendons. This can end up adding too much pressure on the disks of your back or cause a twist or turn in other parts of the body. Therefore, you have to learn how to reduce the risks involved with stretch exercises.

Next up, let's look at the different stretching exercises you can perform.

Chapter 4: Types of Stretching Exercises- Dynamic Stretching

You can have a healthier and more fulfilling life by exercising regularly, especially now that you are over 40. It's important not to forget that stretching too has its benefits to your health.

Most people view stretching only as an exercise to warm up or cool down. But, stretching too has an important role to play in your life.

Do you know there are many types of stretching exercises, each with a different purpose for your body?

Well, when you know the different flexibility techniques in each stretch exercise, you will identify one or more that suits you or incorporate all, or most of them depending on your need or desire.

Let's begin with dynamic stretches in this chapter.

Dynamic Stretches

These stretches are best done before a workout because they loosen your muscles. They involve making movements to warm up your muscles in readiness for a workout, giving your body extra power and muscle flexibility, thereby improving your workout performance.

They are usually similar to the type of activity you will carry out during your workout. For example, if you are a swimmer, exercise your arms in circles, and if you are a runner, your preference will be to jog on the spot before a run.

You can do this type of stretch with any kind of exercise, for example, arm circles, arm swings, spinal rotations, hips circles, lunge, and twist, to name a few.

Since our focus is on stretches for people over 40, find below stretches that will be of help to you:

Arm Swings

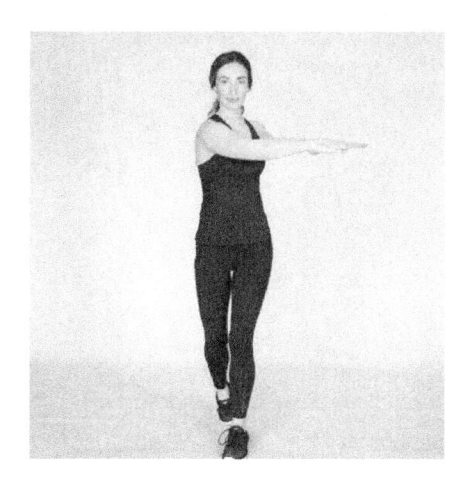

Instructions

1. Stand upright and extend your arms forward shoulder high with your palms facing down.

2. Swing both arms to the left so that your left arm is extended out and your right hand folds at your chest, then swing them to the right side. Keep swinging your arms, remembering your torso should remain straight and only turn your shoulder joints.

3. Do this 5 times on each side.

Spinal Rotations

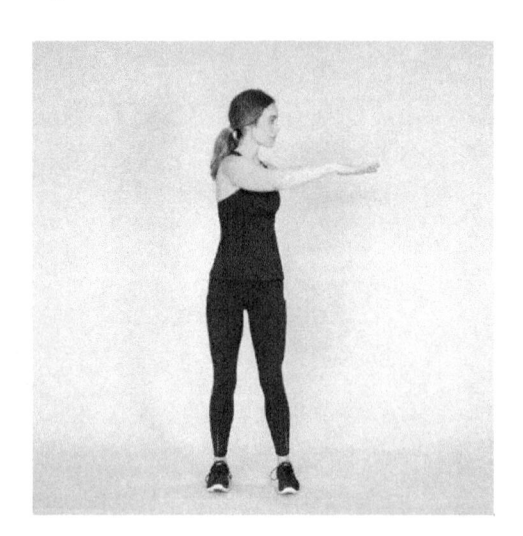

Instructions

1. Standing with your feet shoulder-width apart and with your arms shoulder high, extend both arms outwards to one side.

2. With your torso being still, slowly rotate your body from the right to the left, and move to the other side.

3. Do this 5 to 10 times.

Triceps Circles

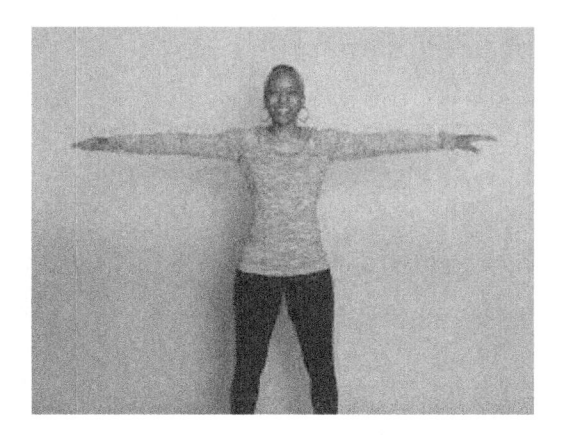

Instructions

1. Hold out your arms to your sides so that they are parallel to the floor with palms facing down.

2. With your arms straight, rotate them forward in small circles for 20 to 30 seconds.

3. Next, rotate the arms backward in small circles for 20 to 30 seconds.

4. Change the direction of your palms to face forward and pulse your arms forwards and then backward for 20 to 30 seconds.

5. Change the direction of your palms again to face up and repeat the pulse movements for 20 to 30 seconds, and then face your palms down and repeat for another 20 to 30 seconds.

6. Do 1 to 3 sets of each of the movements.

Hip Circles

This is a simple stretch that anyone over 40 can begin with. It's great for warming up and slowly increases the flexibility in your hips, helping you to do more intense workouts.

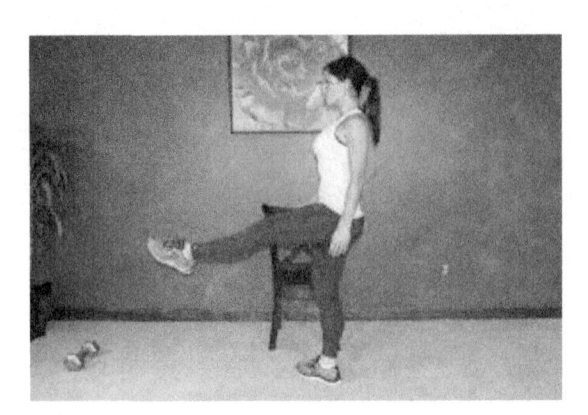

Instructions

1. Stand on one leg, and then hold on to a chair, wall, or countertop for support.

2. Swing the other leg outward in small gentle circles.

3. Do 20 circles on each leg.

4. Do 3 sets on each leg.

Squats

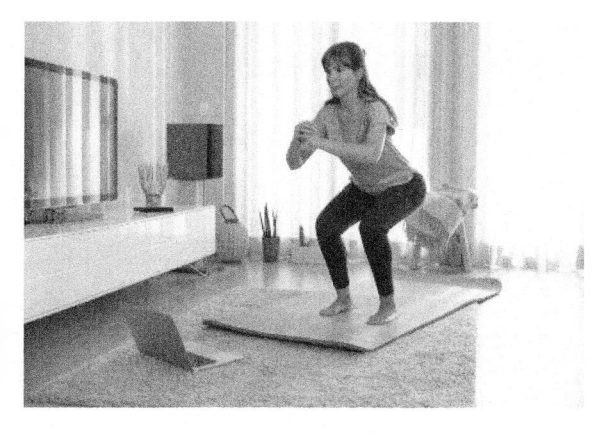

Squats are versatile because they target many muscles in your lower body, including glutes, hamstrings, and quads.

Start with easier squats going down halfway and gradually increase the intensity as your muscles become stronger. As you gain more control over your squats, doing them without pain or aches, you can add weights to intensify your squats further.

Instructions

1. Stand straight having your feet hip-width apart, and face your toes forward or outward slightly to the sides.

2. With your back straight, lower your hips slowly until your thighs are parallel to the floor.

3. Hold that position briefly, making sure your knees do not go beyond your toes.

4. Breathe out and then stand back up.

5. Perform 1 to 3 sets of 12 to 15 repetitions

Side Lunges

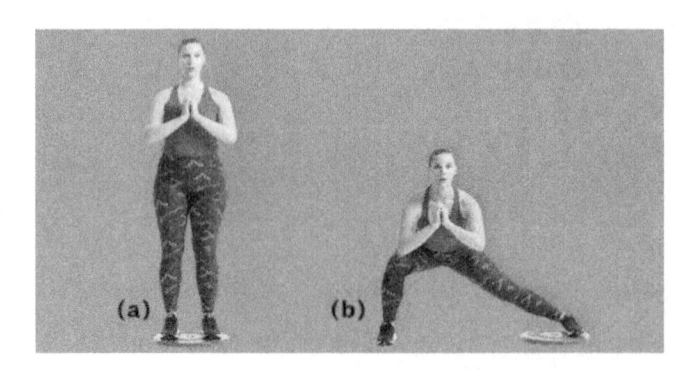

This is another great warm-up exercise for your lower body that strengthens your hips, glutes, and legs. You can perform the easier version of the lunges by going down halfway and gradually progressing to a full lunge.

As your body gets used to this exercise, you can add dumbbells to increase the warm-up intensity.

Instructions

1. Stand upright with your feet hip-width apart.

2. With the right foot firm on the ground, step your left foot forward over to the left.

3. While in this position, squat down as you bend your left leg, keeping your right leg straight.

4. Pause for a few seconds with your left knee over but not beyond the toes. Lift your hips and place back your left foot to the starting position.

5. Do 1 set of 8 to 15 repetitions on the left leg, then switch legs and perform lunges on the right leg.

6. 1 to 3 sets are sufficient enough to warm you up.

Walking Lunge

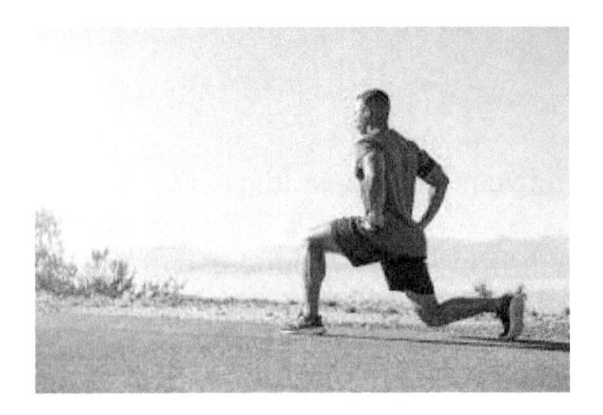

Walking lunge is a good stretching exercise to warm up your body or for your normal flexing exercises.

Instructions

1. Stand upright with your feet hip-width.

2. Straighten your chest up and engage your core and glutes.

3. Hold your waist with your hands on both the right and left sides.

4. Take a big step forward using your right leg and lower your knee until it bends at 90 degrees with your front thigh parallel to the floor.

5. Your left leg should have the knee bent, almost touching the ground at 90 degrees.

6. Go back to the standing position and push your left foot forward into another lunge.

7. Repeat the same motion with each leg you move forward.

Tip

You can make this move a bit more challenging by going down as low as possible with each lunge, all the time keeping your torso upright with an engaged core.

Shoulder Rolls

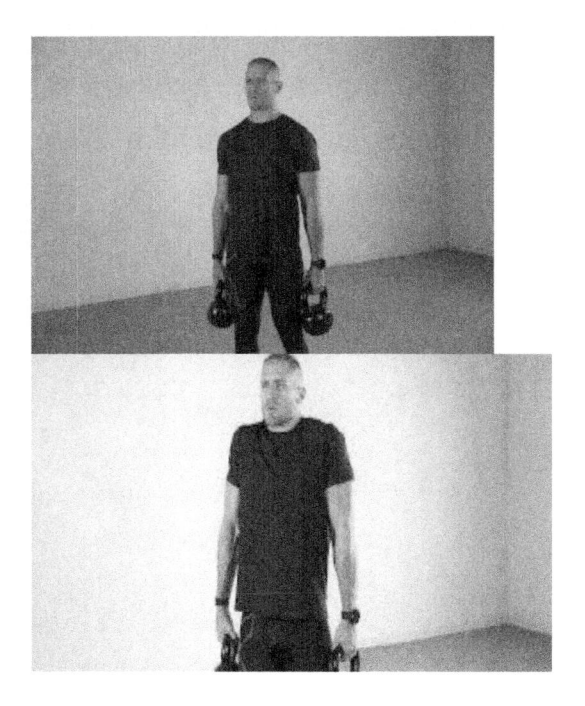

These stretches help to increase the range of motions in your upper back and arms, which you need to reach things that are high up like on a shelf or for sports such as tennis or golf. Your ribs will also open up to help you breathe easier.

Instructions

1. Gently and smoothly roll your shoulders forward in small circles, but make larger circles as your shoulder muscles strengthen. Do this 10 times.

2. Circle in reverse repeat the motion 10 times.

If you tremble during the exercise, stop and rest. Continue the following day, and keep adding more reps as your shoulders get stronger, and eventually add dumbbells to increase the intensity of the stretch.

Walking Knee Hugs

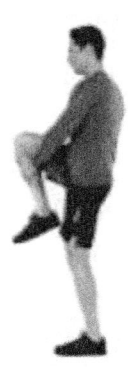

This stretch exercise will improve the mobility in your hip while increasing flexibility in the hamstrings and glutes. You can use it to warm up before your workout.

Instructions:

1. Stand upright with your legs straight and arms hanging loosely in your sides.

2. Move your right knee up as high as is comfortable.

3. Grasp it with both hands and bring it up higher and hug it to your body.

4. Bring it down slowly as you take a step forward.

5. Switch legs and repeat the same motion.

Tip

- Keep your chest up. Also, do not lean too far forward while your shoulders are pulled back during the entire exercise.

- Keep your supporting leg straight throughout the exercise.

Back Pedaling

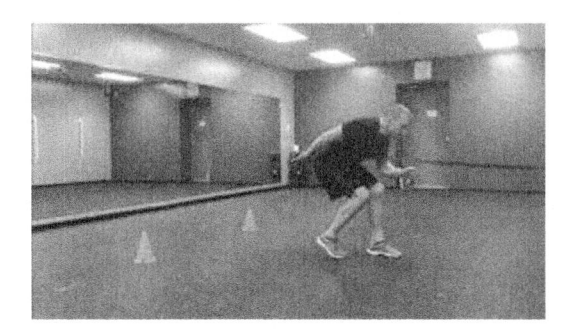

This exercise is good for warming up and targets the quads, calves, hamstrings, and glutes.

Instructions:

1. Keep your hips slightly low in a position similar to a squat.
2. Take small steps backwards.
3. Do this for the distance you desire.

Tips

- Look forward with your head up.
- Walk or run in short quick steps.
- The proper form is to keep your hips low with your chest high.

How Safe Is Dynamic Stretching For You?

Do not undertake any dynamic stretching if you have an injury unless your doctor allows you to. And if you are over 65, you should be more careful when performing these types of stretches.

On the other hand, if you don't have any injuries or your doctor gives you the go-ahead, add these stretches for a good warm-up. You will feel more energized with muscles adequately stretched out and be powerfully ready for a workout.

Are Dynamic Stretches Good For Cooling Down?

Dynamic stretching is amazing for warming up and cannot be done to cool down. This is because they raise the temperature of your body. Cooling down is done to lower the temperature of your body as you wind up your exercises. Instead, static exercises are the best for cooling down, as we will learn more about them in the next chapter.

Chapter 5: Static Stretching

This type of stretching, on the other hand, is done at the end of a workout. You do such stretches by holding a stretch to its maximum point for at least 30 seconds or less, without movement. It aims to loosen your muscles.

These stretches work best if you repeat them at least 5 times before your next stretch exercise and can be done 3 to 5 times a day, or even once a day is enough. They are not necessarily done only after a workout.

And if you do not work out, the stretches are also good for you if your sole purpose is to increase the flexibility of your muscles and joints.

Static stretches can further be divided into two types:

- *Active*: The individual adds more force for greater intensity.

- *Passive*: This is when a force is applied externally, for example, by a partner or a device, to increase intensity.

Below find examples of static stretching that are great after a workout or for improving your flexibility:

Hamstring Stretch When Standing

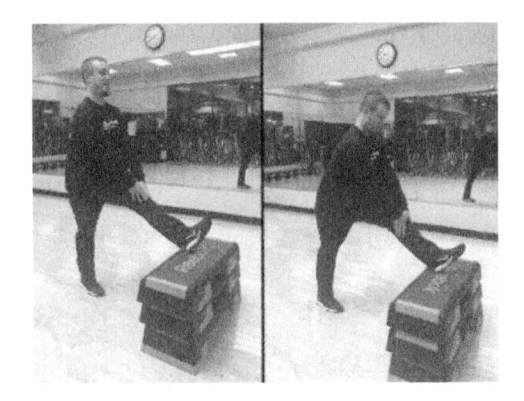

Instructions

1. Stand propped up on one leg in front of the other one.

2. Bend the knee of the leg that's propped up and lean forward from your heaps.

3. To balance your body, place your hands on the bent thigh.

4. If you can't feel the stretch, then lean forward even more or tilt your pelvis forward and hold for 30 seconds.

Hamstring Stretch When Lying Down

This stretch exercise targets the fibers close to your knee.

Instructions

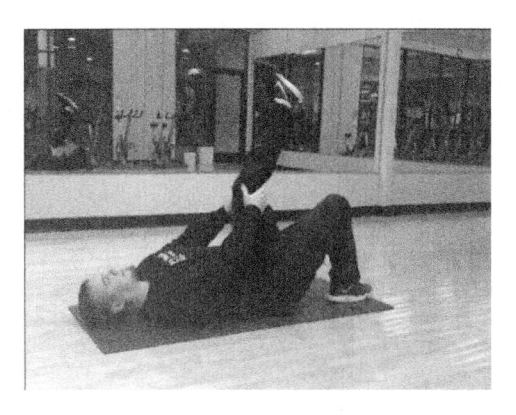

1. Lie down and extend one leg outwards on the ground.

2. Lift up the other leg towards your face, supporting it with your hands.

3. Hold your leg this way for 30 seconds.

4. Change the position of your legs and hold for 30 seconds.

Bent Knee Stretch

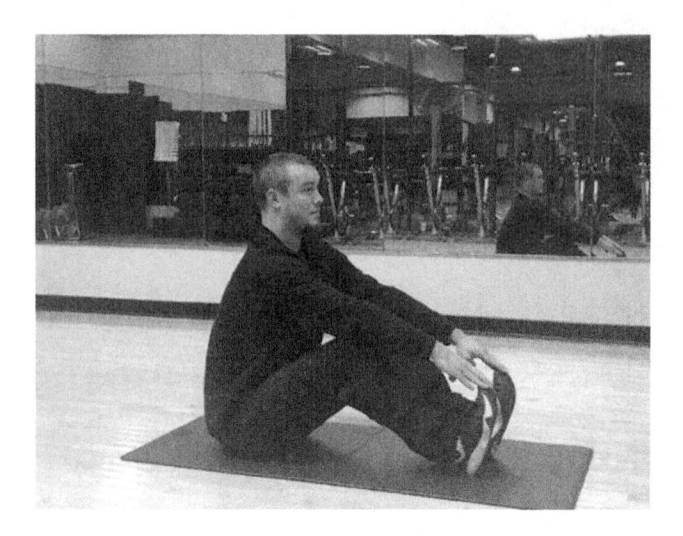

Instructions

1. Sit on the ground, and move your body forward with your legs straight.

2. Touch your toes with your fingers.

3. If it is a little difficult, bend your knees slightly and lean forward, hinging at your hips to touch your toes with your fingertips.

4. Hold this position for 15 to 30 seconds, and repeat 3 to 5 times.

Gradually improve on this stretch by extending your legs a little more straight each time.

Trapezius Stretches

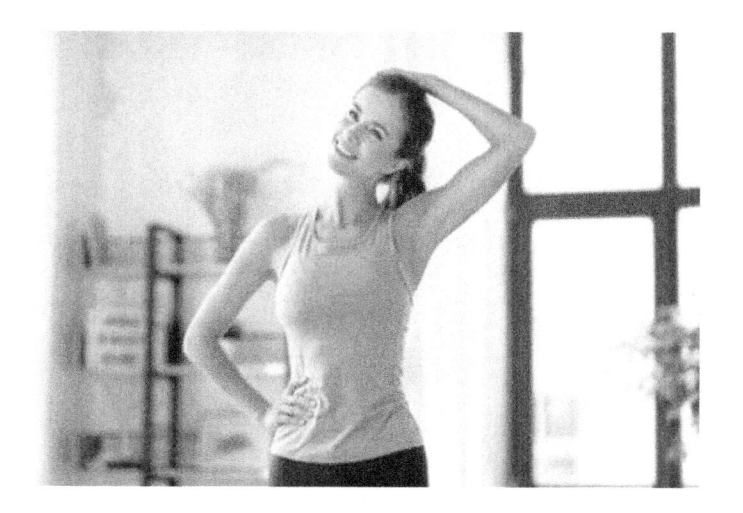

Traps are the muscles, triangular in shape, that hold together your shoulders, top of your back, and the back of your neck. Also, if you spend too much time driving or working on your computer, your trap muscles end up becoming tight and may cause head or neck pain.

Instructions

As you perform this exercise, don't overextend, and if you feel a burning sensation, you're exerting too much pressure.

1. Slowly tilt your head to the right, and hold it for 30 seconds.

2. Next, tilt your head to the left and hold for 30 seconds.

3. To increase the intensity of your stretch, look down at your armpit as you finish this stretch.

Shoulder Reaches

These exercises will make reaching overhead for items in your pantry a lot easier, and also tasks that you do every day.

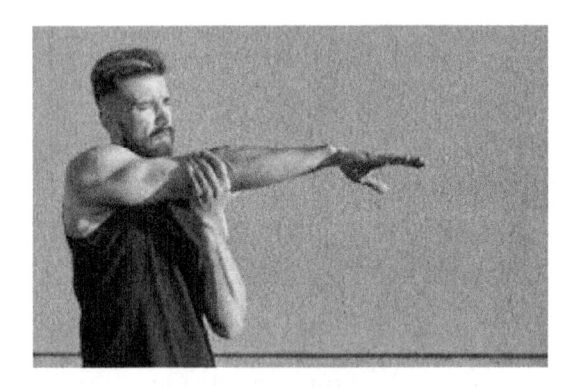

Instructions

1. Extend your left arm straight across your body.

2. With your right hand, grab the back of your left arm and gently pull it to help the stretch on your shoulder.

3. Repeat the stretch, this time on your right arm.

4. Angle your arms slightly down or up. This helps to stretch different sections of your shoulder blades.

Neck Stretches

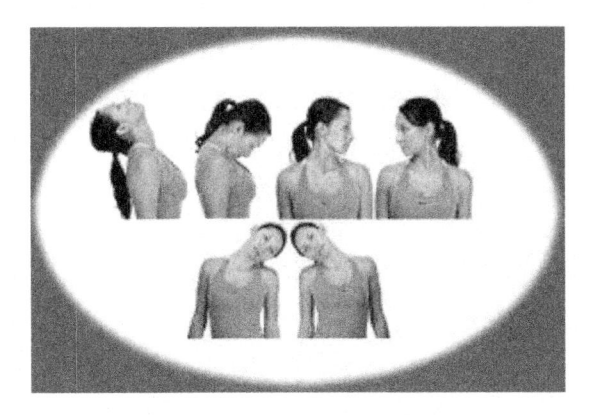

Other than improving strength, flexibility, and relieving tension, neck stretches prevent painful strains or a slouched posture which affects most people as they grow older.

This exercise helps you to stretch all the planes of your neck.

Instructions

1. Look straight ahead and keep your shoulders square.

2. Turn your head slowly to the right as far as you can.

3. Return to starting position and repeat the same motion to your left.

4. Now, turn your head upwards and then down.

5. Next, tilt your head to the right as though you are pinning a phone on your shoulder, and then turn tilt to the left side.

Neck Twist

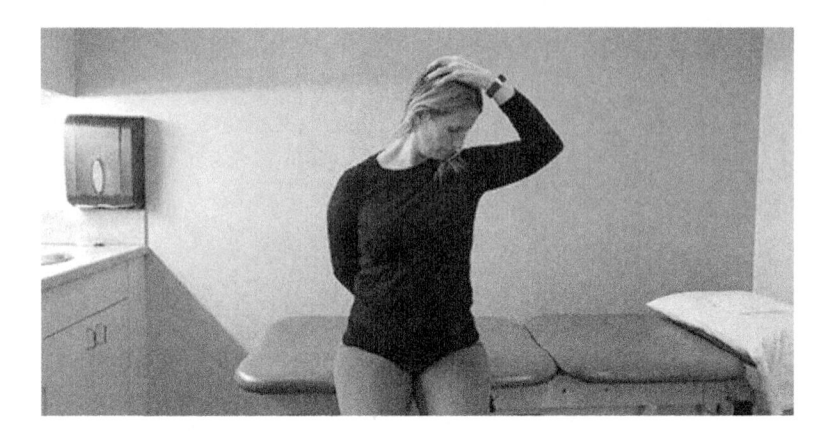

This is a variation of the neck stretch. It targets the scapula and is very helpful if you sit down the whole day, for example, working from your laptop. You gain a much fuller stretch when you place your hands on the tailbone.

Instructions

1. Move your right hand to your back so that it touches your tailbone, ensuring the palm is facing out.

2. Bend your neck to the left, and then turn your head downwards to face your left hip.

3. Guide your head gently toward the hip on your left with your left hand, and hold for 20 to 30 seconds.

4. Repeat the stretch 2 or 3 times on the left.

5. Switch to your right and repeat the stretch exercise.

Quad Stretches

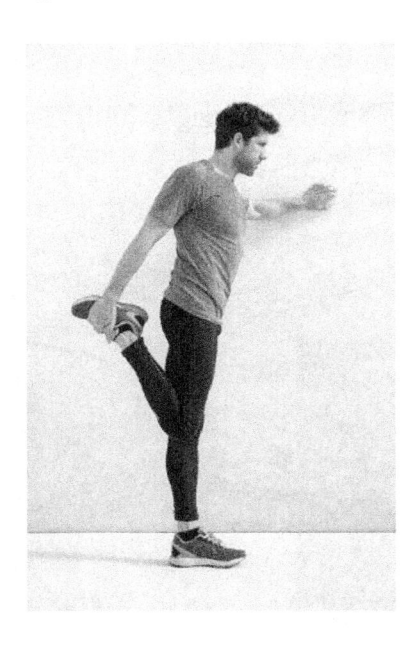

Quadriceps are the large muscles at the top of your thighs that help you sit down or stand up without any help or perform other activities involving your legs. If you sit down for long, they end up becoming tight. Quad stretches can help loosen the muscles for easier leg movement.

Instructions

1. To maintain your balance, stand near a wall or chair or something that you can hold on to.

2. Using your left hand, reach back to grab the top of your left foot.

3. Pull it up towards your butt so that your knee is facing downwards to the ground and not on the side.

4. Change position and do the same to your right foot.

5. Hold for 30 seconds in each stretch.

Lying "T" Twist

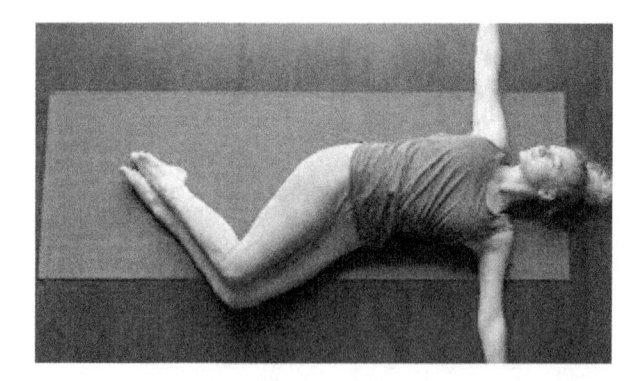

This stretch targets your upper back, spine, and thoracic spine. It opens up the whole spine and helps to loosen the hips and neck.

Instructions

1. Lie on your left side with your arms one on top of the other and extended outwards.

2. Bend your knees together, one on top of the other.

3. Rotate your upper body and head to the right, sliding your right arm across your body to the floor.

4. Hold this "T" position for 10 to 30 seconds, then rotate back to starting position.

5. Repeat 3 to 5 times on the right, then switch sides and repeat the same motion on our left.

Cat-Cow

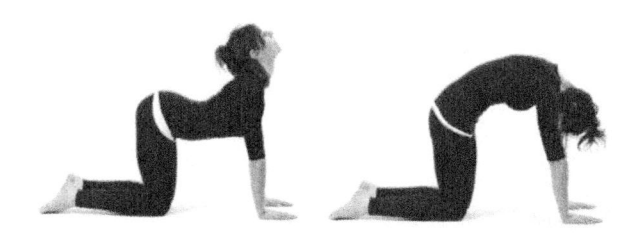

This stretch targets to loosen your lower back, which can stiffen preventing you from sitting, standing, or even walking.

Instructions

1. Go down on your hands and knees, making sure that your hands are under your shoulders and knees under your hips.

2. Arch your back to tighten your abdominal muscles, tucking in your tailbone, and squeezing your butt.

3. Hold this position for 10 to 30 seconds.

4. Release your back and let it sag toward the floor, and allow your tailbone to face upwards, stretching the front of your neck.

5. Hold this position for 10 to 30 seconds.

6. Return to starting position and repeat 5 to 10 times.

Knee to Chest Stretches

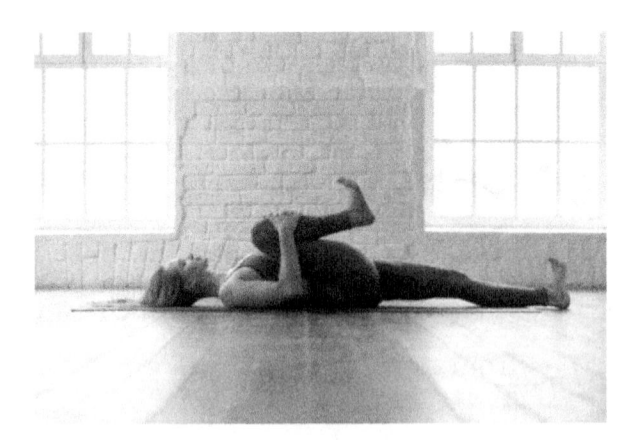

This stretch can help to elongate your lower back and also relieve pain and tension.

Instructions

1. Lie on your back on the floor.

2. Bend the knees and have both feet flat on the ground.

3. Pull one knee using both hands towards your chest.

4. Hold the knee against your chest for 5 seconds, ensuring your abdominal muscles are tight and your spine is pressing against the floor.

5. Return to the starting position.

6. Repeat with the other leg.

Chapter 6: Ballistic Stretching

Ballistic stretching is a type of stretch that involves sudden and fast movements for increased flexibility. It is mostly used by athletes, martial artists, and ballet dancers because they perform extreme motions in their joints. It is also used to rehabilitate to increase joint flexibility and range of movement.

Ballistic stretching is done by bouncing out or into a stretched position by using the stretched muscle as a spring to pull you away from the stretched position. It forces the body to stretch beyond its normal range of motion.

Ballistic stretches use extra force to extend the muscles and the tendons. A good example is bouncing down many times, touching your toes with your fingers. However, your muscles have sensors that tell you how far you can stretch. Therefore, if your sensor senses there is too much tension, it will signal the muscle to pull back to protect your joints from injury.

Ballistic stretching aims to bypass the sensors, allowing your muscles to stretch beyond what is normal.

Is Ballistic Stretching Safe For You?

For most athletes, sportsmen or women, by the time they attain 40, they are no longer fit to continue with their athletic careers. One may be lucky to continue after 40 but rarely does it happen. However, today some men and women have continued their careers well over 40.

For example, Brett Favre[7] who has been playing for the American National Football League, retired at the age of 44 in the year 2010, and Tiger Woods[8] was not slowing down until he was involved in an accident, which has prevented him from playing since then.

Okay, you may never play again for the football or baseball league or race on the track again after clocking 40, but there are other softer sports you can join, such as marathons, cycling, boat adventures, or even weight lifting, to name a few.

---

[7] https://www.menshealth.com/fitness/g28148860/athletes-who-played-after-40/?slide=1

[8] https://www.menshealth.com/fitness/g28148860/athletes-who-played-after-40/?slide=1

Yes, distance running, cycling, or powerlifting over 40 and even 50 is perfectly fine. This is because age is not a major factor in this type of activities. However, be warned to get clearance from your doctor before embarking on any new physical activity.

So, if you are still very active and want to join sports suitable for people over 40, you can do ballistic stretch exercises. But don't forget to start with slower stretches and gradually increase your speed with larger movements.

By making these gradual transitions, your body will become stronger, thereby reducing the risk of an injury. Also, do them correctly to benefit 100% from them.

Continue reading to learn more about the ballistic stretches that you can perform.

Types of Ballistic Stretching

Standing Lunge

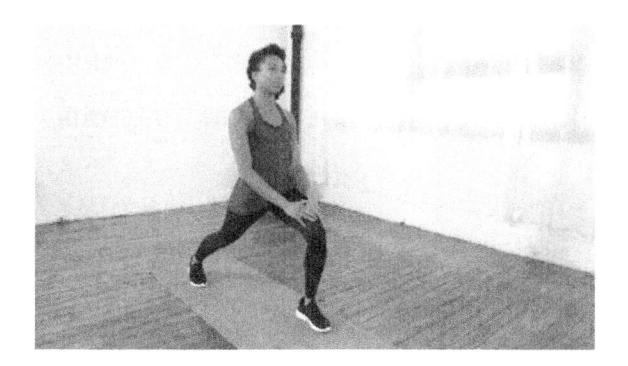

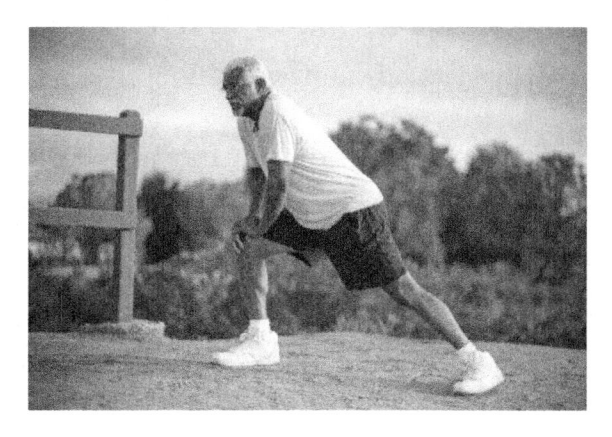

This stretch is great for your quadriceps and glutes muscles. It is an exercise that can be used to warm up or cool down and helps to loosen tight hip muscles due to running, cycling, or sitting down too much.

Be careful that you don't bend your knee too far, bend your back too fast, or sag your hip too much.

Instructions

Warm-up by skipping, jumping, running, or any dynamic exercise that mimics the sport you play. Since this stretch targets the lower half of your body, it's best to perform movements that will warm up the muscles in your inner thighs and groin area.

1. Stand in a split stance with your right leg forward and your left leg backward.

2. Bend the right knee so that you are at a 90-degree angle, putting you in a forward lunge position.

3. Place your hand in your knee that is forward, with relaxed shoulders, even hips, open chest, while looking straight ahead.

4. Press your knee down with your hands, pushing your hips forward until you feel your groin, front of the hip, and left thigh are well-stretched.

5. Hold the move for 20 to 30 seconds.

6. Release the hold and repeat on the left leg.

Mistakes To Avoid

It is possible to hurt yourself while doing these stretches, and therefore it is good to take the necessary precautions as described below:

- Correct Knee Position

Keep the knee that's forward behind your ankle and not in front of it. Also, avoid your knee from turning inward by not arching your back and instead focusing on your back position. Move only through the hip extension and keep the other leg straight behind you to do this.

- Bounce

The bouncing effect of these stretch exercises can tug on the muscle insertion joints and tendons instead of lengthening the muscle. Also, your muscle can tear, making it less flexible and stiff. To prevent this, use slow and smooth movements.

- Exerting Too Much Force When Pressing Down

Just as with bouncing, you can end up putting too much unwanted pressure on your ligaments, insertion joints, and tendons, making you prone to stretching too much and injury.

- Breathing

Ensure you breathe correctly. Exhale when exerting pressure on your knee and stretching your leg backward, and inhale as you relax.

Variations and Modifications

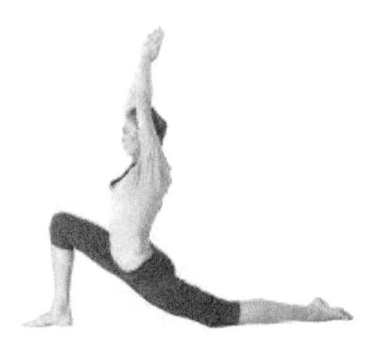

If you wish to move to the advanced version of this ballistic stretch, you can modify it, but be sure you have gained enough strength from the exercise above and that your doctor has checked your health and given you the green light. This stretch can be modified by having the knee in a dropped position.

Instructions

1. Position yourself with a forward lunge, as instructed in step 1 above, and drop your back knee to the ground.

2. Place your hands on the leg that is forward and when you feel your balance is steady, raise your hands and arms above your head while looking forward.

3. Press your hips downwards and forward. You should feel a strain in your thigh, groin, hip, and torso.

4. Hold your stretch in this position for 20 to 30 seconds.

5. Release and repeat the same motion on the other leg.

Tip

As you increase your stretch, make sure that you do not let your back hip sag. Your hips should be centered, activating your abdominal and pelvic floor. This will protect your lower back from any injury.

Stand Toe Stretch

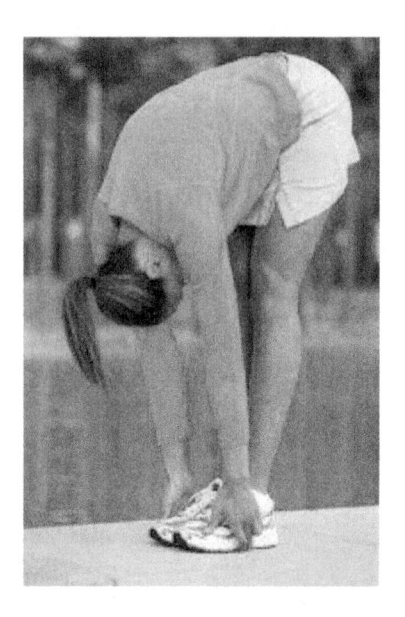

If done correctly, this exercise not only stretches your hamstrings but also stretches and works your shoulders, butt, calves, and abdominals.

Instructions

1. Stand upright. Have your feet shoulder-width apart and your toes facing forward.

2. With straight legs and knees bent slightly, extend your arms down on your sides.

3. Bend forward at your torso, keeping your body loose, and then let your fingers hang down towards your toes.

4. Hold this position for 20 seconds.

5. Stand up and repeat again.

Tips

- Reach only as far as your hamstrings can stretch. It is okay if, in the beginning, you are unable to touch your toes. Gradually, you may be able to touch your toes.

- Keep your knees slightly bent throughout the exercise to reduce the risk of injury.

- You can include variations of this stretch by adding different types of toe-touching exercises.

Seated Toe Stretch

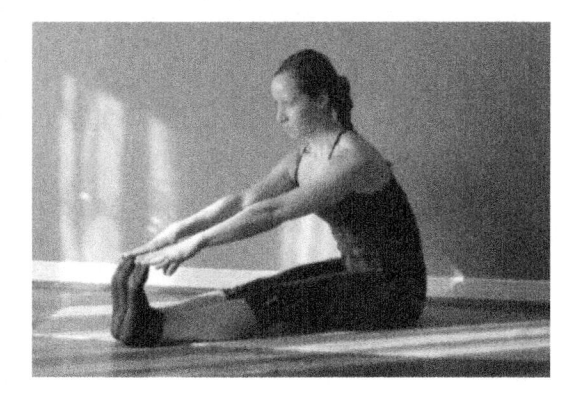

This exercise targets your thighs, calves, and shins. To start this stretch, sit down with an upright body, your legs extended out and your toes pointing to the ceiling, and do not bend your knees. Make sure your head is aligned to your spine.

Instructions

1. Place your hands at the top of your thighs.

2. Stabilize your spine by stiffening your abdominal muscles.

3. Bend forward from your hips and exhale as you do so, and extend your hands so that your hands touch your ankles and finally your toes.

4. All the time, maintain a flat back, avoiding to round your back. To avoid bending your back, move from your hips and not your lower back. You should feel a stretch in your calves, hamstrings, and lower and middle back.

5. Continue bending as you reach forwards to touch your toes until you feel a point of tension.

6. Hold this position for 15 to 30 seconds.

7. Relax and then return to starting position and repeat 2 to 4 times.

Tips

- You may decide to hold your position by only grasping your ankles instead of your toes.

- You can perform a variation of this stretch by performing slower, more controlled movements and completing 1 set of 5 to 10 repetitions, holding each stretch for 1 to 2 seconds.

- To prevent injury, do not extend beyond the point of tension, and do not round your back but keep it flat.

Side Arm swings

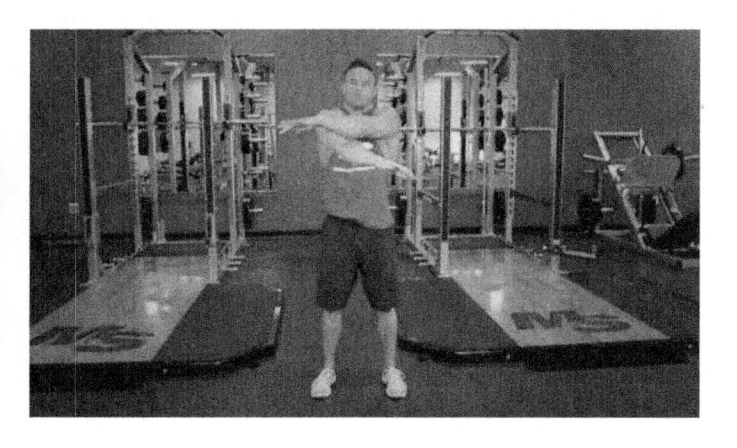

These are great exercises for warming up and stretching your shoulders, chest, arms, and upper back and preparing your muscles, joints, and tendons for a workout. It provides a great boost to your cardio exercises and increases your flexibility.

Instructions

1. Stand upright with your knees bent slightly and your feet shoulder-width apart.

2. Stretch out your arms horizontally to the sides.

3. Cross your arms in front of your chest and then quickly stretch them out as far back as you can.

4. Repeat this forth and back movement until you complete a set.

Correct Form and Breathing

Keep your back straight, tightening your abs. Your face should face forward as you slowly breathe while you move your muscles. Make sure that you also swing your arms in smooth and steady motions.

Variations and Modifications

An excellent variation of the sidearm swing is the overhead arm swing, which can also be used as a warm-up exercise.

Instructions

1. Stand upright with your feet shoulder-width apart. Now, slightly bend your knees and keep your back straight.

2. Swing your arms forward, over your head, backward, and upward to the starting position.

3. Repeat 6 to 10 times.

Leg Swings

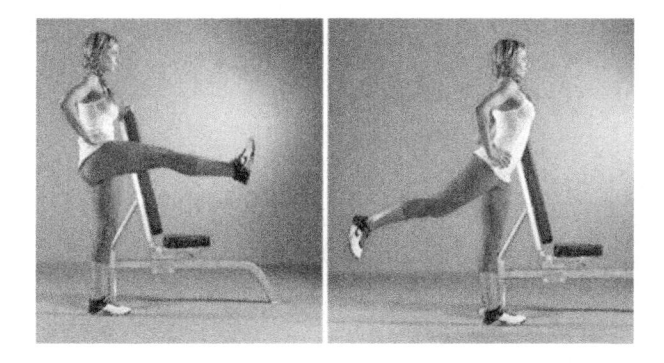

This stretch targets your hip muscles, calves, quads, and hamstrings. It is a great exercise for warming up and stretching your hip muscles and hip joints. The motion helps you to prevent injuries and reduce pain in your hip area.

Instructions

1. Stand straight with your feet hip-width apart and use your left hand to hold onto a wall, chair, or something appropriate.

2. Place your right hand on your waist.

3. Slowly swing the right leg forward and backward. Swing them as high as you can in both directions.

4. Switch legs and repeat the range motions to complete a set.

5. Repeat 10 to 20 times

Correct Form and Breathing

Keep your upper body stable, your abs tight, and have a steady deep breathing pattern. Use your muscles to swing your legs back and forth.

Shoulder Rotations

This is an advanced form of shoulder rotations. It is very useful for athletes who constantly put pressure on their shoulder joints, such as through baseball, handball, volleyball, tennis, and other activities involving throwing or hitting. It improves muscle flexibility in the chest and shoulders.

To improve your shoulder range of motions, follow the instructions below.

Instructions

1. Stand straight with your arms extended to your sides, and straighten them.

2. Face your palms upwards to the ceiling and flex your elbows.

3. Rotate your shoulders forward 10 to 20 times.

4. Repeat backward 10 to 20 times.

5. Start with a few repetitions, slowly increasing them.

Chapter 7: Isometric Stretching

Isometric stretching involves contracting a muscle or group of muscles without moving. It is a form of static stretching that may require an outside force to assist in stretching. Your partner can help to provide resistance to a particular muscle, or you can use a wall or anything else that's suitable. For example, your partner can hold your leg up as you try to force your leg back down.

It is more effective than active or passive stretching and is an excellent method to develop your flexibility very fast. It is performed by first assuming a static position, then applying tension on a muscle for 10 to 15 seconds, and then relaxing it for at least 20 seconds.

Because an isometric stretch is done in one position without motion, it will improve the strength of one particular muscle. To strengthen many muscles in your body, you would have to include different types of isometric stretching targeting those particular muscles.

Other than a general improvement on your flexibility, it is also an excellent stretch if you have an injury that makes movement painful. For instance, if you have an injured rotator cuff, your physical therapist or doctor can recommend isometric stretches involving those muscles that help to stabilize and increase your shoulder strength.

Let's delve into 4 ways in which isometric stretch can be used to improve your health.

1. Healing From Injury

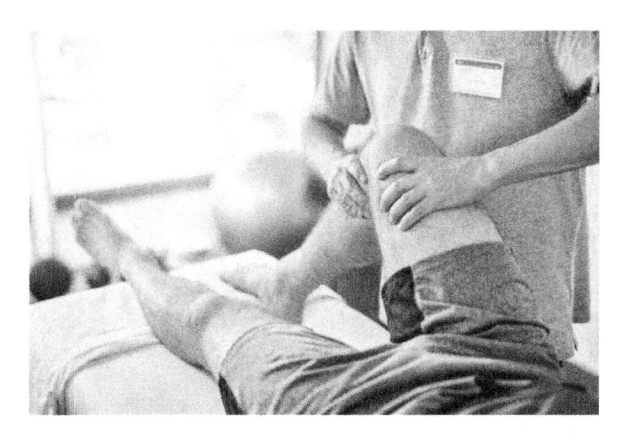

If you've suffered a knee or shoulder injury, the first stretch treatment is normally isometric. For example, your physical therapist or doctor will recommend that you contract your quads for a few seconds and then release them. You will be asked to do this several times.

For your knee to heal properly, your doctor will prescribe between 10 to 30 seconds of contracting your quads at different angles including, fully bent leg, leg bent at 90 degrees, and when your leg is straight.

This approach does not allow any movement in your joints, making it very safe. Your doctor may also request extra force from a trained therapist to assist you with isometric contractions and releases.

2. Improving Your Posture

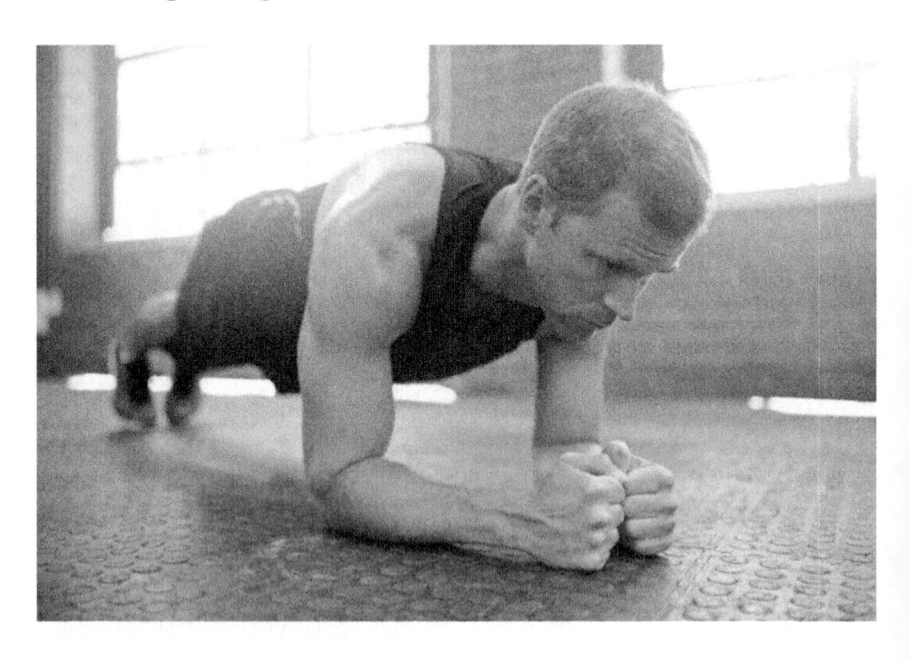

The primary goal of your muscles is to assist you with movement. However, some muscles can be strengthened by not moving. Your core muscles are a great beneficiary of these stretches and are best done when stationary.

If you spend a lot of your time behind a computer and feel your posture has been affected, these isometric stretch exercises are good for you, such as planks, side planks, leg raises, hollow holds, or deadlifts. They work by holding your torso and contracting your core muscles.

Doing this strengthens the muscles that form your posture, mainly in your lower back and mid-back. After a few of these stretches, you will experience improved posture.

Another exercise you can do to improve your posture is by raising your arms to the level of your eyes while standing upright with feet shoulder-width apart and then contracting your shoulder blades so that they come together. Hold for 30 seconds, and then release. After a few of these exercises, you will feel stronger in your shoulders.

3. Improving Muscle Strength

It is true that for your muscles to become stronger, you need to move them. Isometric contractions, in particular, are equally effective in increasing muscle strength. For example, if you contract your quads while lying down or seated, they will get stronger.

Use this exercise to your advantage, as you can do them almost anywhere.

Are you at the store waiting for your turn at the till? You have a good chance to squeeze your shoulder blades several times, holding them for a few seconds before releasing them. Do as many as you can, and by the time you reach the till, you will be feeling great!

How about ladies who love a firm butt? You can do these when seated, lying down, or also at the store. Contract your glutes for a few seconds, release them, and then repeat. Perform several reps, and in no time, you will feel your butt is firmer.

Below are isometric stretching exercises that are simple and can be done anywhere:

Plank

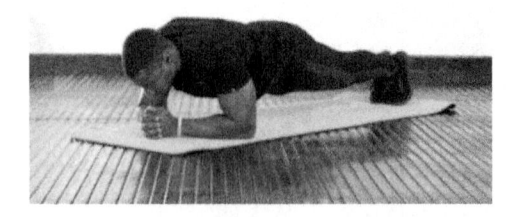

Performing a plank is similar to doing a press-up but without moving your arms. As a beginner, or if you have a shoulder problem, you can start by placing your forearms and elbows on the floor. The other more advanced plank is to straighten out your arms and elbows out under your shoulders. Use a soft mat to cushion your elbows, which will help you keep your body grounded during the plank exercise.

Instructions

1. Get on all your fours and put your feet together with your body straight from head to heels, ensuring your hands are in line with your shoulders.

2. Hold your torso so that it does not touch the floor, and do not lift your hips too high.

3. Tense your core muscles holding your body in position and clench your glutes.

4. Hold this position until you feel tired.

Correct Form of Doing The Plank

- Hold your spine in a neutral position, including your head. To do this correctly, imagine your spine is a straight pole, keeping your head and neck in line with your back.

  Don't crank your neck up such that it bends down, or your overall form and strength will be interfered with.

- Hold your hips in line with your spine as you keep checking your posture, making sure you do not lift your hips up and don't dip them either.

- Lock your knees, keeping your legs straight.

- If you struggle with this plank, you can start with your knees on the floor and slowly build up to a full plank.

As you work towards improving your plank, remember to:

- Tense your abs so that you can engage them. This ensures that you engage your core correctly.

- Check your posture throughout the exercise because you are likely to drop or raise your hips. When you can't hold the plank any longer, then stop and rest.

- Time your plank so that you can check your progress. Start with 20 to 30 seconds, and if you wish to, you can build it from here, though it's good to note that if you can hold a plank for 2 minutes, then it's a sign that you have significantly strengthened your core.

- Engage your glutes as well, which will help you build as much strength as you can.

How Many Times Should You Plank?

If you have a weak back, start with many planks that last only a short time, and 3 times in a day is adequate. As you become stronger, you can do fewer sets that last a little longer than you did previously. 3 to 5 times per week is enough.

Finally, do not strain your muscles if you get too tired.

Lateral shoulder raise

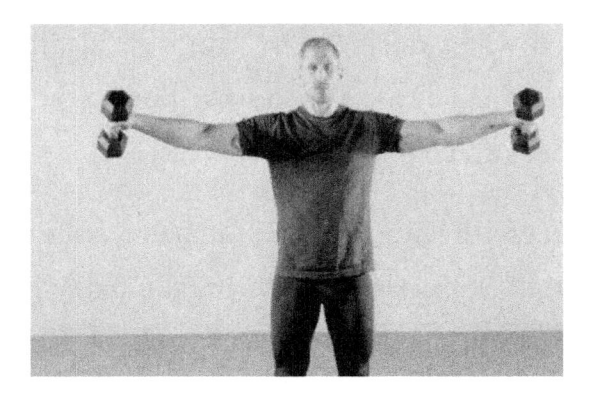

This stretch exercise targets the shoulder muscles, upper back, arms, and chest. You'll need some dumbbells.

Instructions

1. Hold a set of dumbbells with your hands, and stand straight.

2. Face your palms down, and then lift the dumbbells by raising your arms outwards to your sides until your elbows are at the same height as your shoulders.

3. Pause in this position, and then lower your arms slowly back to the starting point.

4. Do sets of 3 and repeat between 8 and 12 times.

How to Breathe and Properly Do the Exercise

Keep your core engaged when raising your arms, ensuring your back is straight. Inhale as you bring down the dumbbells with your knees and elbows slightly bent.

You can perform this exercise without the dumbbells, but if you do use them, you'll be strengthening the middle part of your shoulders. Not forgetting that your upper back, chest, and arms become much stronger.

Bridge

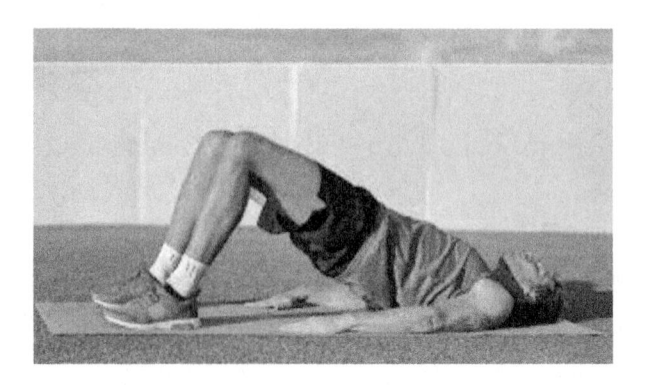

A bridge stretch targets your glutes, hamstrings, and core muscles. It's great for spine stabilization.

Instructions

1. Lie on your back and bend your knees at 45 degrees angle, with your hands on your sides.

2. Lift your hips off the floor while your back is straight, and pause.

3. Return to starting position, and repeat the motion.

4. Do 2 to 3 sets and repeat 12 to 16 times.

Proper Technique and Breathing

Press down your heels to lift your hips, and keep your glutes and core tight. Exhale when lifting your butt off the ground, and inhale as you return to starting position.

Hollow-Body Hold

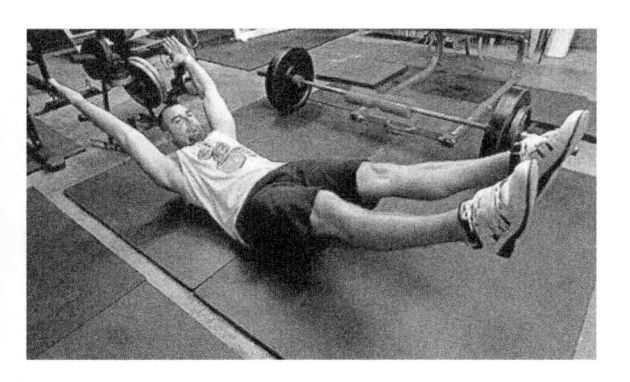

If you want to increase the strength in your abs and core body muscles, then this is the exercise for you. Start by holding your body for a few seconds, and gradually increase to more seconds.

Do these stretches exercise as follows:

1. Lie on your back, making sure it is flat.

2. Contract your abs such that it's like you are pulling your belly button downwards to the floor while your arms and legs are held straight outwards from your body.

3. Raise your shoulders and legs slowly from the floor while the lower back is touching the floor.

4. Your goal is to maintain your hold to the lowest position possible without your arms and legs touching the floor and without your lower back touching the floor.

Tips

- Ensure your butt and abs are tight during your hold.

- Begin this exercise by first raising your arms and legs and holding them 1 to 2 feet off the floor for 10 seconds, and as you get stronger, you'll be holding for close to 30 seconds.

Calf Leg Raise

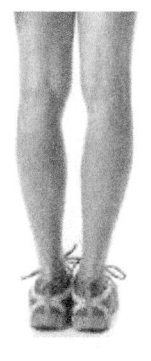

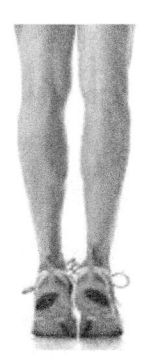

This is an easy stretch exercise to perform that strengthens your calves.

Instructions

1. Raise both legs by lifting your body off the ground using your heels.

2. Go as high as you can, and when you can't go any further, hold this position for 10 to 30 seconds.

3. As your body can hold without stressing too much, you can add an extra 30 seconds.

Wall Sit

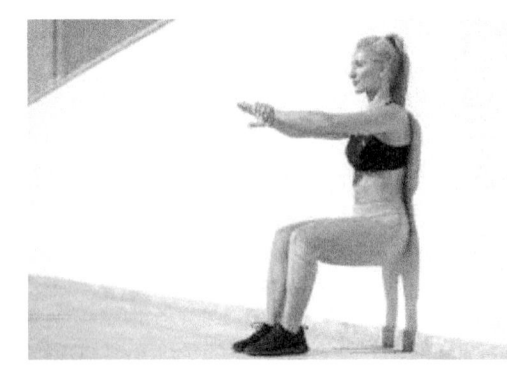

You can perform this exercise almost anywhere, for as long as you are near a wall. It's a great exercise for your glutes, calves, and quads.

Instructions

1. With your feet hip-width apart and hands by your sides, stand with your back against the wall.

2. Slide down the wall until your knees and hips are bent at 90 degrees, as your butt and shoulders touch the wall.

3. Hold this position and stop when the strain is uncomfortable for you.

Leg Extension

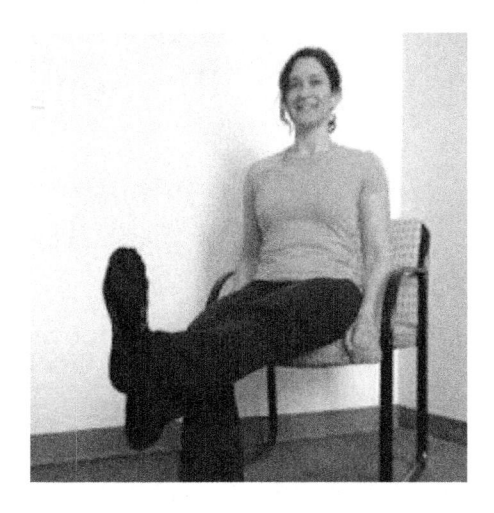

Leg extensions are the answer to strengthen your thigh muscles and improve the mobility in your knees.

Instructions

1. Sit on a chair with your butt firmly against the back of the chair, and hands on the chair, and both feet flat on the ground.

2. Slowly extend one leg in front of you as you engage your quads until your leg is straight.

3. Stay in this position for about 10 to 30 seconds, and then lower the leg to the starting position.

4. Switch legs and repeat the motions 8 to 12 times.

Chapter 8: PNF (Proprioceptive Neuromuscular Facilitation) Stretching

PNF stretching is an advanced type of flexibility exercise that involves the stretching and contraction of muscles. This technique was initially used as a clinical rehabilitation move and spread into gyms because it is believed to be effective.

It was designed to increase activity, tone, and relax muscles; it is now popular with athletics to increase muscle flexibility. They are normally performed with a partner, using both passive (concentric) and active (isometric) muscle actions.

Although PNF stretching is thought to be superior to other stretching methods, it is sometimes seen as impractical because most stretches require a partner or physical therapist.

Types of PNF Stretching

PNF stretching uses both the passive (concentric) and active (isometric) stretches to apply tension on the muscle being stretched. In other words, a muscle is stretched and contracted at the same time.

There are three types of PNF stretches

- Hold-relax

- Contract-relax

- Hold-relax with agonist contraction

These are three phases of each technique. The first phase involves a pre-stretch of 10 seconds. The second and third phases differ in each technique.

1. Hold-Relax

To achieve this technique, begin with a passive pre-stretch, which will create a mild discomfort, and hold it at this point for close to 10 seconds. A good example is the hamstring stretch.

Hold your right leg up and contract it without moving while your partner applies force on your hip by pushing your leg towards your chest. Hold this for 6 seconds, as seen in the figure below.

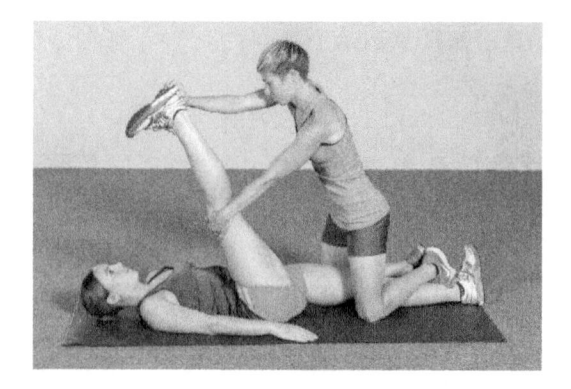

You will then relax, and your partner will apply a greater force to your hip as seen in the figure below.

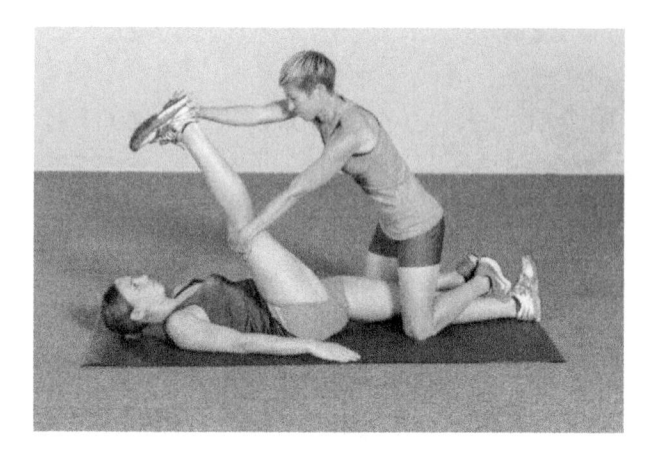

2. Contract-Relax

This technique is almost like the hold-relax technique, but in this technique, there is movement involved. As in the example of hamstring stretch, you will resist your leg from being pushed towards your chest and instead push it towards the floor while your partner applies pressure so that your leg moves to your chest.

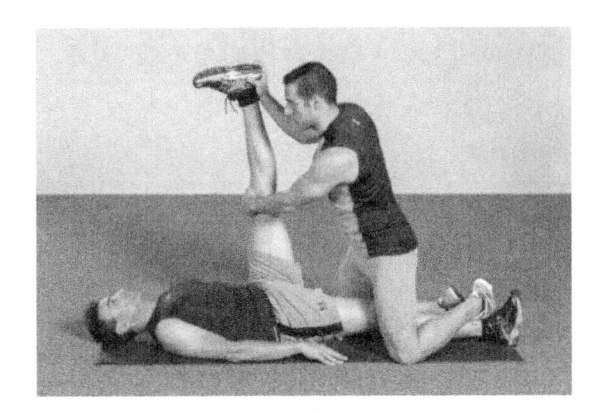

3. Hold-Relax With Agonist Contraction

This is a technique in which your partner applies force on your muscle, and you apply force in the same direction. For example, in a hamstring stretch, you push in the same direction your partner is pushing.

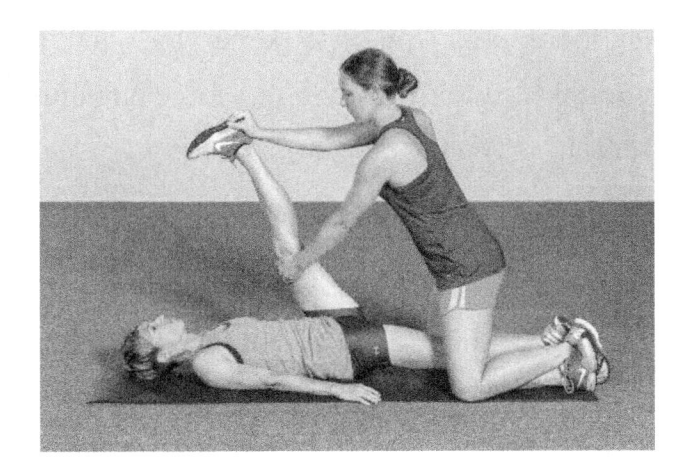

Precautions to Take As You Perform PNF Stretches

Whichever PNF technique you decide to perform, there are some precautions you need to take as sometimes you can add undue stress on the targeted muscle/s, which can increase the risk of injury on your soft tissue.

Basically:

- Do not apply maximum force as you stretch and contract your muscles. This technique works best by applying gentle pressure on both the stretches and contractions.

- The smaller the muscle, the less force you should apply. For example, do not apply much force on your shoulder or neck, as you would your hamstring.

- Remember to warm up before you perform any stretch, including PNF stretch exercises. You will benefit more when you warm up to increase your temperature in preparation for the stretch.

Chapter 9: How to Start Your Stretching Routine

To improve your flexibility and experience the full benefits of stretching and see actual results, you will need a regular stretching routine. If you have never stretched before and this is your first time, you will need to start with light stretch exercises that are slow without using too much force.

You will gain momentum as your body gets used to these exercises until you start performing them much more easily.

Next, you need to perform your stretch exercises correctly to avoid the risk of injuries and gain maximum benefit to your muscles and general body wellness.

You also need to know that you can stretch any time during the day. It is up to you to come up with suitable times so that you do not miss a day of stretching.

Workout Stretches

On the days you exercise, purpose to perform dynamic stretches for 5 to 10 minutes before your workout. Follow with static or PNF stretching for 5 to 10 minutes after working out.

Non-Exercise Stretches

On the days you will not be exercising, you still need to plan a routine to exercise for at least 5 to 10 minutes. It will reduce tightness and pain in your muscles and improve your flexibility.

It will be important to focus on the main areas of your body that are concerned with mobility, such as quadriceps, hamstrings, calves, and hip flexors. For your upper body, stretching your lower back, neck, and shoulders will strengthen the muscles in those areas.

You can begin a simple stretch routine that works your full body. Start with the top part of your body and gradually downwards so that you do not miss working any muscle or group of muscles.

As you begin your daily stretch routine, you may find it difficult, especially if you have a busy schedule. However, just by setting aside 10 to 15 minutes each day in the morning or before you go to bed in the evening, then you are well on your way to a more flexible body.

Below is an example of a stretch routine that you can begin with and develop further as you get stronger:

Neck Roll

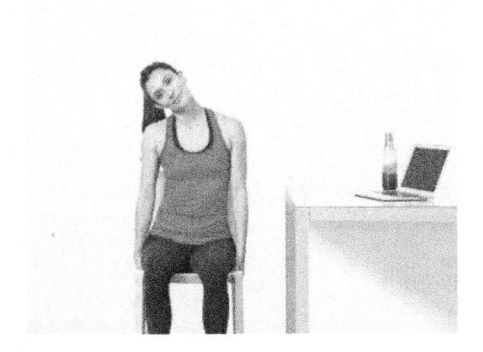

Instructions

1. Stand straight. Have your feet shoulder-width apart with your arms loosely on your side. You could also sit on a chair.

2. Move your head so that your chin is facing your chest.

3. Gently roll your head clockwise and complete a full rotation that should take about 7 seconds.

4. Take a 5 seconds rest and then roll your head gently anticlockwise using the same motion.

5. Repeat 3 times on each side.

Shoulder Roll

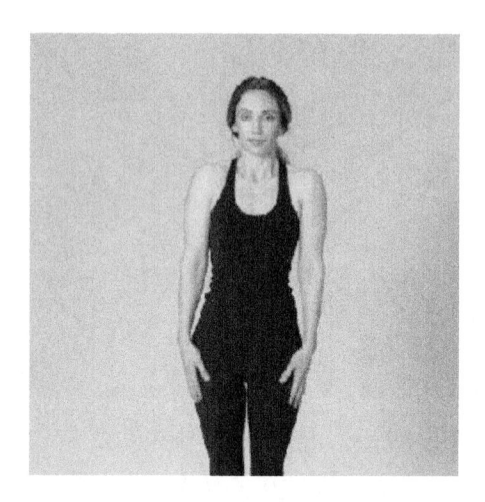

Instructions

1. Stand upright with arms on your sides.

2. Slowly raise your shoulders and then roll them backward five times in a circular motion, making sure your arms are not bent.

3. Repeat the same motion forwards.

4. Do 2 repetitions for the backward and forward shoulder roll.

Triceps Stretch Behind Your Head

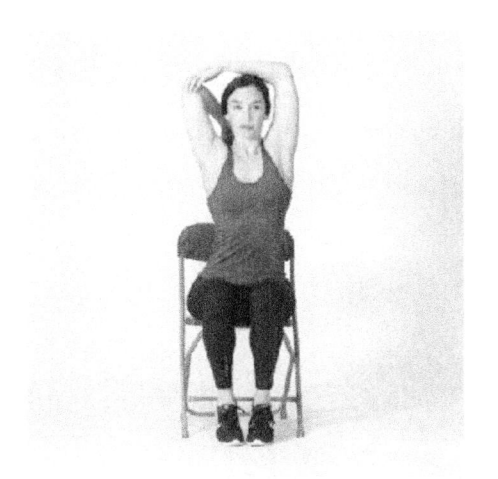

Instructions

1. Raise your left arm upwards, with your elbow next to your head.

2. Bend the elbow, dropping your hand behind your neck.

3. With your right hand, hold the upper left arm at the elbow behind your neck.

4. Gently press the elbow so that you push your left hand down your back.

5. Hold for 10 seconds, and rest for 5 seconds before moving to your right arm and repeating the same motion.

6. Do 3 sets on each arm.

Hip Rotation

1. With your feet shoulder-width apart while standing upright, place your hands on your hips.

2. Move your hips forward, and rotate them clockwise 3 times.

3. Bring back your hips back to starting position, and repeat the same motion anticlockwise.

Standing Hamstring Stretch

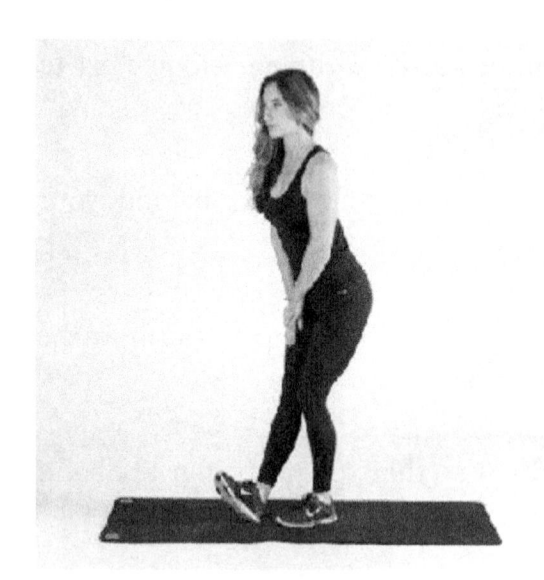

1. Stand upright, keeping your left foot flat on the ground. Bend the left knee slightly and extend your right leg forward.

2. Flex your right foot with your heel on the ground and toes facing upwards.

3. Place the hands on your left thigh and slightly lean forward, raising the right toes.

4. Hold it there for 20 seconds. Relax for about 10 seconds, and repeat the same movement on your other leg.

5. Do 3 repetitions on each leg.

Quads Stretch

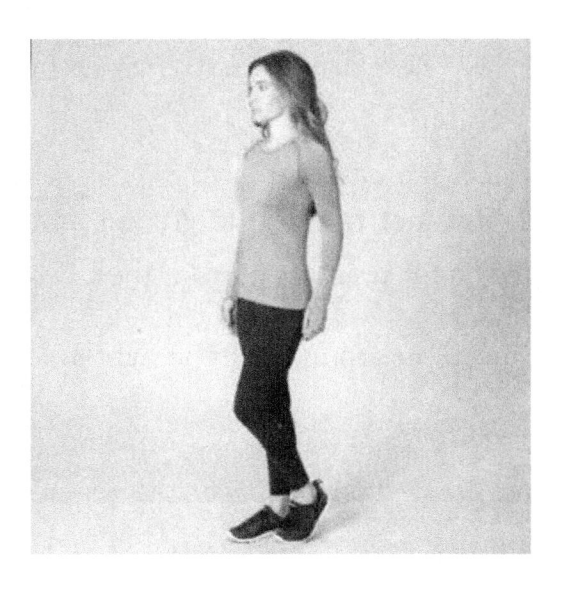

1. Stand upright, and for balance, hold onto a wall or solid structure with your right hand.

2. Stand with your right leg straight with the foot flat on the ground.

3. Bend your left knee so that your left foot is behind your right leg.

4. Gently press your foot, squeezing your left butt while keeping the knees and hips in line.

5. Hold for 30 seconds.

6. Rest for 20 seconds, and then repeat on the opposite leg

7. Do 3 repetitions on each leg.

Rolling Your Ankle

1. Standing with your left foot flat on the ground and your right heel raised, apply pressure on your toes.

2. With your toes firmly on the ground, roll the right foot in the clockwise direction.

3. Do 10 repetitions, and then repeat the same movements anticlockwise.

Child's Pose

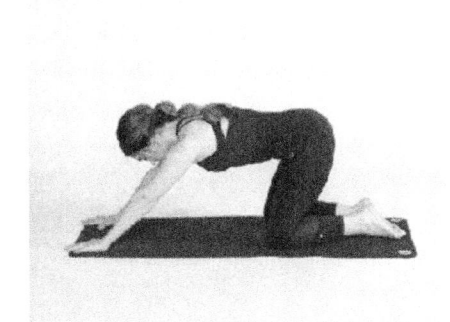

1. This is a yoga position that you can do as you finalize your stretch routine.

2. Kneel down with your hands on the ground and toes facing backward. The top part of your feet should be lying flat on the ground.

3. Move backward so that you end up sitting on your heels.

4. While in this position, push your butt backward and then lower your chest to the floor as you stretch your arms forwards.

5. Hold this stretch for 30 seconds.

6. Rest for 10 seconds and then repeat 3 times.

A daily stretching routine can improve both your mental and physical aspects. Stretching is a superb way to keep your muscles loose, hence lowering the risk of strains and sprains.

However, do not forget to consult with a doctor or physical therapist if you feel pain when stretching, as this could mean there is an underlying problem.

Chapter 10: Safety Tips and Overcoming Risks

Like any other exercise, stretching can be risky to your health because of injuries that can occur while performing the exercises. There are safety precautions you have to observe to prevent injuries, including:

- If you have an injury, perform stretches only as directed by your doctor.

- Suppose you have an injury for too long. In that case, you may have to consider using the services of a physical therapist or medical specialist who can design a stretching routine suitable for you.

- If you have limitations to how far you can physically be active, consult with your doctor to prescribe exercises that will safely help you increase your flexibility.

Irrespective of your fitness capabilities, there are some standard safety tips that you need to follow:

- Avoid stretches that involve bouncing of muscles. For example, ballistic stretches are mainly done by bouncing and are very helpful at focusing on a single muscle or group of muscles. Athletes use this lot to help them strengthen particular muscles depending on the sport they do.

These exercises can cause injuries to your muscles, especially if you are a beginner and you are not yet strong. If you want to perform these stretch exercises, it is highly recommended to consult with your doctor or physical therapist.

- Don't stretch beyond what you are comfortable with. While it is perfectly normal to feel the tension in your muscle when stretching, you should not feel pain. If you start to feel pain or it hurts, stop the stretch.

- Don't over-exercise. All forms of exercise put a strain on your muscles. Performing the stretch exercises many times on the same muscle, and sometimes many times in a day, you risk causing damage to the muscles.

- It is always advisable to warm up before any physical activity such as a workout or stretch exercise. This means that you should never attempt to stretch when your muscles are cold because stretching becomes more difficult.

A warm-up of 5 to 10 minutes, such as jogging or walking, is good for warming up your body in readiness for your exercise.

When to See a Doctor

Keeping fit is a healthy lifestyle. However, it is good to see your doctor first before you start any stretch exercise.

Especially if you have been inactive for some time, it is highly recommended that you see a doctor to check your body. You will either be allowed to exercise or be given guidelines on which exercises to begin with and how to do them, depending on the health issues you may be having.

If you have certain health conditions, you definitely need to see a doctor before beginning any stretch regimen. These conditions include:

- High blood pressure
- Ongoing treatment for cancer, or you've recently finished cancer treatment
- Arthritis
- Kidney disease
- Type 1 and 2 diabetes

- Heart disease

Seeing a doctor incase of any of the above conditions helps avoid any potential risks or dangers as a result of stretching. Also, if you have symptoms related to lung, heart, or any other serious disease, you need to see a doctor. These are symptoms such as:

- Pain in the lower part of your leg that goes away when you rest.
- A pronounced or rapid heartbeat even when you are at rest.
- Swelling of your ankles, which happens mostly at night.
- Shortness of breath after mild exercise, when resting, or when lying down.
- Lightheadedness, fainting, or dizziness after much exertion after a workout.
- Discomfort or pain in your chest, arms, jaw, neck while resting or during a workout.

The above list of symptoms is not exhaustive and is a guideline to inform you that if you have any type of symptom that presents as serious, consult with your doctor.

Overall, as indicated above, or if in doubt, then it is advisable to see a doctor. This way, you will plan for an exercise program suitable for you, reducing potential risks to your health.

Conclusion

Being over 40 does not mean you cannot slow down the aging process. You can do so through stretching to loosen your tight joints and making your muscles firm to help you continue with your everyday activities with ease.

You can begin with stretch exercises that do not require heavy exertion but rather light movements like shoulder, ankle, and leg rotations. These are mostly done before a stretch exercise, but can also be performed any time during the day, even if you do not plan to stretch.

There are many types of stretching, each with its purpose, such as dynamic stretches used for warming up before a stretch exercise and static stretch, which is mainly done after a workout. Others include ballistic stretching, which is excellent for athletes, isometric stretching that concentrates on certain muscles or a group of muscles. And finally, PNF stretching, which is an advanced form of stretching that involves both stretching and contracting the muscles.

For stretching to benefit you and produce results, you have to do it correctly. Therefore take into consideration the elements of a good stretch. Also, before you plan any stretching regimen, you need to consult with your doctor, more so if you have not been active for some time, if you have an underlying condition, or you simply want to be sure that you are healthy enough to start stretching exercises.

The benefits of stretching are immense and can improve your health tremendously. Incorporate it as your lifestyle and enjoy growing old gracefully.

Good luck!

PS: I'd like your feedback. If you are happy with this book, please leave a review on Amazon.

Please leave a review for this book on Amazon by visiting the page below:

https://amzn.to/2VMR5qr

Printed in Great Britain
by Amazon